MW01259050

Sex:

The Best Guide to Last Longer in Bed

Recover Your Sex Life and Improve Love and Romance on Your Relationship

(Sex Guide, Sex Health, Marriage and Sex)

2nd Edition

Bruce Maxwell

Disclaimer

This book is intended for informational purposes only. It is not designed to treat, cure, or diagnose any disease, health problem or medical condition, and then it is up to the reader to consult a healthcare professional.

This book is not a substitute for medical advice. The author is not to be held liable for any injury the reader may endure as a result of reading this book.

Bruce Maxwell

Table of Contents

Bruce Maxwell

Introduction

I'm glad you have take the chance to purchase "The best guide to last longer in bed, how to overcome premature ejaculation, become the best lover and give more power and health to your penis naturally". I really believe that you will find great information here, despite this being a short book.

There are lots of reasons why you might not be lasting as long as you would like in bed and not all of them are going to be your fault. The reasons range from health – stress, medical problems, disease or illness – to diet, weight, overall health and, in some cases just plain over-excitement!

There is always a way around everything and there are ways to teach yourself to hold back a little, to wait. At the end of the day, sex is not a race; it should be pleasurable for both parties, not a competition to see who can get to the end first.

This title is intended to give you proven steps and techniques on how to improve your lover skills. This book was not created only for the man who has premature ejaculation problems, but for anyone who wants *more* and wants to take advantage of a maximized manliness.

Put these strategies into action and you won't get disappointed with the results. Commit yourself to your improvement, **you're worth it.**

Chapter 1
Keep the End in Mind

This book is intended to groom men to be Casanovas of the times. It will not discuss matters on luring women, nor will it tell you of ways to keep a woman. What this book focuses on is taking care of oneself.

When a person is cared for and loved, it will then be very easy to reciprocate such affection. It may be emotionally or sexually. In this case, the focus will be on a man's sexual aspect. Various aspects will be discussed.

You will learn the knowledge you need to be able to take good care of yourself. Later on, familiarization with the common problem of premature ejaculation will be done. It is a common problem among men of all ages. Furthermore, the care of the reproductive system will be discussed, and so will the things men need to avoid to build up a healthy and satisfying sexual life.

Each time a man sets his mind to a task, he must keep his goal in mind. The goal of this book is to develop a man into the best lover a woman could have. This means not shortchanging her and instead giving her due pleasure.

For a man, this may cause him to exude more confidence, knowing that he is able to satisfy his partner while at the same time satisfying himself. This may play a big role in a relationship.

While reading this book, keep in mind that sexual health is tackled through a multi-factorial approach. Many different factors contribute to keeping the male reproductive system at its finest condition. All topics discussed in this book point to that means to be able to reach the goal of Lasting Longer in Bed: How to Overcome Premature Ejaculation, Become a Best Lover, and Give More Power and Health to Your Penis Naturally

Let's take a look at what your goals should be. Obviously, your main aim is to be able to last longer in bed and know that you have satisfied your woman. Many couples simply don't feel satisfied for one reason – because they don't communicate and neither knows what the other's goal is when it comes to sex. So, let's take a look at five goals of sex that will all have a relationship, direct or otherwise, on how long you last in bed:

Goal 1 – Orgasm

This is the one goal that most people seem to be after, the be all and end all of the sex. Hopefully, both of you will achieve orgasm and then, that's it, all over until the next time. That's not a good goal for someone who suffers from premature ejaculation - nobody will end up satisfied and it will all be over quicker than it began.

Why is orgasm a goal in sex? Is it a measure of whether the sex was pleasurable or not? If it is, it shouldn't be. Think back to times when you never orgasmed but you had some amazing sex. Think back to when the sex was brilliant but the orgasm was something of a damp squib and of course, we've all had the "one" that came out of nowhere after what can only be described as mediocre sex.

Sometimes, that orgasm just isn't going to happen, mostly for women but sometimes for men as well. Not every woman will have an orgasm every time but that doesn't mean you've failed, it doesn't mean you should give up and it doesn't mean you are a bad lover. If you spend all your time focusing on the orgasm as the end goal, you might find it's too much pressure and you just won't get there.

It isn't a bad thing to have the orgasm as a goal of sex. Some people do just want a quickie and there isn't a thing wrong with that. Just don't make it that way every time otherwise you will never learn to stay the pace in bed.

Goal 2 – Pleasure

So, think back to that night where you had the most amazing sex but neither of you was focusing on the orgasm. Everything just gelled, everything flowed like it should and you both just went for it. You may not even have ended up having an orgasm but I bet it all felt good anyway.

That is because you were focusing on, most likely subconsciously, the pleasure of the sex. There isn't any need to chase that orgasm, there isn't any need to get over the finishing line first but there is a need to experience true, out of this world, pleasure.

So why don't we do this all the time? Certainly, if you are not focusing on reaching the finishing post, you could find that you can last for some considerable time in bed. Unfortunately, life tends to get in the way and sex begins to be seen as nothing more than a stress reliever – we all know that a good orgasm can knock stress on the head. Or, you don't have a great deal of time, you have to be up early and it's getting late – you need your sleep.

It isn't that you are not enjoying sex, you just don't have the time to, there's too much else going on. It is important that, while a quickie is fine on occasion, you find the time to spend in bed.

Forget about the orgasm, forget about everything else that is going on in your life, just lose yourself in the pleasure.

Goal 3 – Exploration

Did you spot an article on the internet or in a magazine, showcasing a position that you might like to try? Maybe it was about the G-Spot and you want to know more! On some nights, forget about the orgasm, forget about racing to the finishing post. Instead, concentrate on what you read, what you wanted to explore. You could even forget about the pleasure aspect; your main goal here is to learn, to try out new things. But, take it slowly, take your time about things. And, you know what? So what if you reach orgasm too early? It doesn't mean you have to stop. Carry on exploring, carry on learning and carry on enjoying yourself.

Goal 4 – Procreation

Obviously, if this is your goal, then the game changes slightly. It can be a very stressful experience, having sex purely to procreate, especially when you have to do it at certain times of the month. The pressure is on you to perform and, if you are having trouble, it just makes things a whole lot worse. The romance disappears, the spontaneity s gone and there is no excitement anymore.

Set aside time to have sex with your partner without proration being the goal, just to have fun and enjoy yourself. Remember that sex is meant to be fun and not a chore that you have to perform.

Goal 5 – Connection

When you've been away from your woman for a while or you just haven't been connecting with one another properly, even if you see each other every day, when you finally do get it together, the sex is going to be one of two things – fast and furious or slow and tender. It should be tender, slow, lots of touching, as if you've just seen the eighth wonder of the world and reverently worshipping her. It should be lots of kissing, lots of looking at one another. It shouldn't be rushed – it's just the two of you and the whole word is outside and is of no consequence.

These are just five of the main goals that people have or should have in sexual relationships. Of course, you can also count exercise and comfort as goals. Where the problems occur is when you both have different goals. If for example, your woman wants comfort, and you, because you find it very difficult to last very long in bed, are going for the orgasm as the end goal, things are bound to go wrong.

Talk to each other. Find out, every single time you have sex, what your goals are. Believe me, they will be different every time and the only way you are going to be in tune with one another is to talk. Communication is the real key to any relationship and to most sexual encounters. This is even more true if you don't find it very easy to last longer than a few minute; instead of leaving her there puzzled, upset and unsatisfied, talk to her, tell her what the problem is, what your fears are. Then, and only then, can she begin to understand and start to help you.

Bruce Maxwell

Chapter 2

The Superstar

Building an impressive performance in bed is like grooming a movie star. It always starts with the talent. You get to know him, his strengths and weaknesses, as well as what gets him excited, what makes him tick, and of course, what he's made of.

So, gentlemen, we start by getting relatively familiar with the star of the show, the reproductive system.

Many, if not all, adolescent boys only recognize the two external parts of the reproductive system, which are the penis and the scrotum. This is understandable as these two parts alone can give you the pleasure most desired. However, hidden inside the male genitalia are a series of complex mechanisms that contribute to the overall well-being and overall ecstasy derived from sex.

The penile head is the seat of sexual pleasure, as is the clitoris in women. Its shaft is made up of spongy material and filled with blood during sexual stimulation that it enlarges and becomes rigid. It is the main tool by which a male is to deliver his sperm to a female.

At the root of the penis hangs the scrotum. It houses the testes, where the factory for sperm production is found—a man's genetic heritage. This is connected to a set of tubules where the immature sperm stay for approximately 20 days before they are mature enough to travel forth.

The sperm is otherwise known as the **gamete** or male sex cell. Each testicle is capable of producing at least 4 million brand new sperm every single hour! The testicles or testes hang outside of the body for a very good reason. For sperm to develop normally, they must be kept at a temperature that is approximately two degrees cooler than body temperature. It can take between four and six weeks before sperm matures and they do this while they are traveling from the testes to the to a tube that is coiled on the outside of the testes, known as the **epididymis.** Sperm is often called tadpoles because that's what they look like and the use their little tails to propel themselves while the head of each sperm is where the genetic material is housed.

The main character, of course, always has his support staff—the accessory glands. Their role is to produce the semen, where the sperm is mixed in. They activate the little tadpoles, giving them nutrition to travel through the acidic environment of a woman's body.

When sexually stimulated, an initial release of a thick, clear mucus-like substance is made from the male organ's supporting staff. This is to cleanse the passageway of any remnants of acidic urine. The passageway of urine and sperm converge into only one duct. The passage of urine and semen, however, cannot happen at the same time. There is a valve regulating the entrance to the duct such that during intercourse, it prevents the entrance of urine. The same is true during urination. The entrance releasing the sperm is closed.

Shortly thereafter, a series of wave-like movements and muscle contractions occur to propel the vitamin C-filled semen into the ejaculatory tubes, where soon, they find their release into their promised land.

How this happens is that smooth muscles start to contract during sex and push the mature sperm from the epididymis through the **vas deferens**, a long tube inside the body, just underneath your bladder. The sperm is them mixed up with a fluid from the seminal vesicles, full of nutrients, and a milky secretion that comes from the prostate gland. Mixed together, this is what we call semen and that is responsible for doing three things:

- Providing an environment of watery fluid for the sperm to swim in once they exit the body
- Providing the necessary nutrients for the sperm – vitamin C, amino acid, and fructose
- Protecting the sperm by neutralizing the acids that are found in the usual tract in the receiving female

As soon as the semen has been made, it will pass through your urethra, inside the penis, and exit the body through the tiny slit at the top of the penis in the process we all know as ejaculation. On average, one ejaculate will contain about one teaspoon of this seminal fluid and only one percent of that will be sperm itself.

This release of steaming hot sexual tension cannot be done, however, without the act of sex itself—or the simulation of it. This entails the penetration of the penis into the vagina, position notwithstanding. Friction is then created to build up tension which results in an orgasm.

The superstar is healthy and in good shape. All that is needed now is an effective supporting star to give that ultimate performance: the pubococcygeal muscle or PC muscle.

This muscle located in the pelvic floor of the human hip appears to be a sheet hanging from the pubic bone to the tail bone. It controls the sphincters, or the valve which releases or holds in the urine or feces, during urination and defecation. When in good shape, this muscle contracts to enhance sensations while having intercourse.

The PC muscle is the muscle that you squeeze while running to the restroom when your bladder is full. *To identify the muscle, stop the flow of your urine midstream. The muscle you contract to do this is your PC muscle.* Furthermore, you may touch the star when you insert your finger into your anus, feeling around the sphincter as you contract the muscle.

A healthy package, an efficient supporting staff, and a competent actor will ensure that you are well on your way to last longer in bed.

10 Things You Never Knew about The Male Sex Organ

As a bit of fun, these are ten things that you might not have known about the male sex organ. These facts are courtesy of Dr. Trina Read, an author and sex therapist, who has this to say about lovemaking versus intimacy:

"Too often people assume that the word 'intimacy' has to do solely with sex: saying things like, 'Let's get intimate tonight.' She also sad that she is often asked, when she goes on some shows, if she can use the word "intimacy" in place of "sex", just to make sure kids can watch it. To that, she says: *"Intimacy is in fact a deeply shared connection to another human being. Sex just*

happens to be an easy segue to get to intimacy. We have intimate moments all the time with people who we are closest to: children, parents, friends, spouse."

And, just in case you were wondering why women tend to stay awake longer than a man after sex – a man's brain will be flooded with a sleepy hormone called serotonin while the woman's brain is the recipient of a flood of epinephrine, which wakes her up.

Fact 1 – Semen is very fast

Did yo know that semen leaves the man's body at pretty much the same speed rate as a city bus but can reach dizzy speeds of 43 miles per hour? That will depend on how long it has been since the last sexual encounter but, suffice it to say, be careful if you are just playing around after a long stint without any form of sexual gratification

Fact 2 – Testicles are not the same size

Mostly it is the left testicle that isn't quite the same, not as "pert" as the right one., although left-handed men, sometimes the opposite is true

Fact 3 – You don't get the same amount of semen every time

The average amount of semen expelled during sex between one teaspoon and a tablespoon but this amount can change – more the first time and then, for every subsequent encounter, the amount lowers

Fact 4 – The glans and the frenulum are the sensitive parts

The glans is the head of the penis and the frenulum is the skin, on the underside of the penis just below the head.

Fact 5 – Blood flow has an effect on the sex organ

When a man becomes aroused or get cold because of a temperature change, the cremaster muscle will raise the testicles. The pens itself contains only spongy tissue, no bone, and no muscle so erections rely solely on blood flow into it, with exit veins constricting to hold the erection in place by stopping the blood from flowing out again

Fact 6 – Men can have "dry" orgasms

What this means is that nothing is ejaculated, usually because he has recently ejaculated and there just isn't anything left to come out. Taoist belief is that this is the way to build up the male essence and lets the man absorb the female essence, part of a healthy libido! Those who recommend Tantric sex say that this is the best way to experience true intimacy as a pathway to "spiritual ecstasy".

Fact Seven – Enhancements for male libido aren't always what they are cracked up to be

If a man is going to take libido enhancements, he has to actually be turned on if they are going to work. The way they work is that they increase the flow of blood to the penis; they are not designed to enhance the actual sexual desire. Perhaps the most famous of all these enhancements is Viagra, the little blue pill that is supposed to work wonders – it doesn't always work and you should really only take it under direction from your doctor

Fact Eight – Kegel exercises are not just for men

I will talk a little more about kegel exercises later on in this book but, contrary to popular belief they are not just for men. Women can also benefit from them because both sexes have the kegel muscles – they are located between the pubic and tail bone and will involuntarily contract during sex. Kegel exercises are perfect for strengthening up the ending.

Fact Nine – Patience truly is a virtue

Especially with sex. A man aged around 65 will take anywhere from 12 to 24 hours for a repeat erection, on average – some will take longer while others will take less time. Every man is different mostly dependent on age and health, so don't be disappointed if you can't manage sex twice on a night like you used to

Fact 10 – Women aren't the only ones with a G-spot

One of most common misconceptions is that only women have a G-spot but men do too. So where is it? It's the prostate gland, a gland the shape of a walnut that contains pretty much the largest concentration of the liquid

Bruce Maxwell

Chapter 3

Keep Your Enemy Closer

Keep your friends close, and your enemies closer. Men rarely talk about premature ejaculation because this is a direct insult to their ego. But as self-help anonymous groups dictate, the first step to solving the problem is admitting you have a problem.

Premature ejaculation is spilling semen way before you or your partner intended. This may happen shortly after penile penetration into the vagina. In some cases, this happens even before penetration is performed. This may cause dissatisfaction to both partners and when no improvement is made, it may certainly be a cause of problems.

Men of all ages are affected by premature ejaculation. Most men, if not all, at one point in their lives, may have gone through this problem. The complaints seem to arise from different situations and there is no definite cause for the condition. It is believed that the cause is multi-factorial.

Some theories say that it is caused by initial overstimulation and lack of control of it. Others say that it may be due to a lack of practice or long periods without intercourse.

Psychological causes may also play a part. This includes experiences of previous trauma and loss of confidence due to frequent experiences of premature ejaculation.

There may also be relational causes, such as less attraction to your partner. A male who also feels inferior to his partner, for whatever reason, may also exhibit these conditions.

Spiritual and social influences may also cause someone of high moral standards to view sex as a sinful activity and cause sexual problems.

The physical aspect of premature ejaculation is the very last to be investigated once all the aforementioned causes have been treated or ruled out. Physical causes of premature ejaculation are rare. Deeper evaluation may reveal problems in the reproductive system or the urinary tract.

With prolonged premature ejaculation, more severe erectile dysfunctions may occur. As with most conditions, early detection is the key. The earlier you set forth to solve the problem, the earlier treatments and solutions can be made.

The important thing you should note is that premature ejaculation is not a life-long condition. It is transient as it is treatable. Through diligence, healthy living, and proper care of your package, you will be able to control the situation.

Treatments and Drugs

Like most things there are certain options for treatment for premature ejaculation. It isn't the end of the world and it doesn't mean that you have any serious medical conditions. Only a very tiny number of people can actually attribute premature ejaculation to a medical complaint but if you are at all uncertain, you should go and see your doctor. Treatment options include topical anesthetics, behavioral techniques, counseling and oral medications. Do keep in mind that the results are not going to be instant, except perhaps in the case of Viagra or other similar medications, and it may take time to find the right treatment for you.

Behavioral Techniques

Therapy may be prescribed and this will involve a number of simple steps for you take, steps like masturbating a couple of hours before you are going to have sex. This can help you to slow down ejaculation during the actual act and help you to last longer. You may also be told that you should avoid actual penetration during sex for a while and concentrate your efforts on other types of sex play. That can help to remove a lot of the pressure from sex as you won't be expected to "perform" as it were.

Pause and Squeeze

This technique is often touted by doctors as a god way of holding things back and it will involve your partner. It works like this:

- You should begin sex as you would normally, making sure your penis is stimulated almost to the point of ejaculation
- At that point, your woman will need to squeeze your penis at the end where the head and shaft join one another. She should hold the squeeze for a few seconds, until you lose the urge to ejaculate
- Once she releases you from the squeeze, wait another 30 seconds then resume your foreplay. You might find that your penis loses some of its rigidity when it is squeezed but don't worry; once you get back down to the pleasure, your erection will return!
- Again, when you get to the point of ejaculation, your partner will squeeze again

This should be repeated as many times as you feel necessary until you get to the stage where you can actually penetrate your partner without immediate ejaculation taking place. After a while of doing this, you will get to grips, if you'll pardon the pun, with knowing how to stop yourself ejaculating straight away and you won't need to continue with this technique

Topical Anesthetic

These are sprays and creams that contain an agent like prilocaine and lidocaine, agents that cause numbing. If your doctor recommends this course of action, you will have to apply the cream or spray a little while before you are going to have sex, so that the sensation is reduced and you can delay your ejaculation. You can purchase these products over the counter but it is best to go to your doctor.

While topical anesthetics can be effective, they do have the potential for side effects. Some users have reported a decrease in sexual pleasure and a loss of sensitivity and, in other cases, the woman has reported feeling the same thing. Also, if you have to apply these creams a short while before you have sex, it means that you are having to plan it and that means the fun is gone, there is no spontaneity anymore.

Oral Medication

There are a few oral medications that can help to slow down an orgasm from happening but many of them are not actually approved by the FDA for the treatment of premature ejaculation. However, that doesn't stop them from being used and include antidepressants, phophodiesterae-5 inhibitors, and analgesics.

These might be prescribed for daily use or to be taken on-demand, and they may also be prescribed as part of a plan that includes other treatments as well.

- **Antidepressants** – Some men have had great success with using these to delay things a little, simply because one of the side effects of most antidepressants is a delay in orgasm. The most common ones prescribed for this purpose are of the serotonin reuptake inhibitor family – Zoloft, Paxil, Prozac or Sarafem. If these are not successful in helping to slow down the time it takes you to ejaculate, you may well be prescribed Anafranil, or clomipramine – a tricyclic antidepressant. Unfortunately, the possible side effects of nausea, a dry mouth, feeling drowsy and a decrease in libido (not what you want) may be enough to put you off taking this one

- **Analgesics** – Perhaps the better known of these is Tramadol, normally prescribed as a painkiller with a side effect of delaying ejaculation. It may only be given to you AFTER the above SSRI medication has been tried and failed Again, the side effect may be unpleasant enough to make you not want to take it.

- **Phosphodiesterase-5 Inhibitors** – These medications are generally used as a way of treating erectile dysfunction but can also help in cases of premature ejaculation and include Viagra, Revatio, Cialis, Adcirca, Staxyn, and Levitra. Side effects may include a flushing of the face, headaches, temporary changes to your vision and nasal congestion

Counselling

Also called Talk Therapy, counseling involves you sitting down with a mental health provider and talking about your experiences and your relationships. The idea behind this is that it can help to cut down the amount of anxiety you feel about your performance in bed and to help you cope better with stress. This is normally used in conjunction with drug therapy.

A Personal Story – How I Dealt with Premature Ejaculation

This the story of how one man overcame premature ejaculation; we'll call him Sam for the sake of preserving his identity. Hopefully, his story will help you to see that you too can overcome this troubling situation. It might also go some way towards showing you that, truly, you are not alone. More men that you realize suffer from premature ejaculation; they just don't talk about it, mainly because of the perceived embarrassment and the stress it causes. Without wasting any more time, let's hear what Sam has to say

The loss of my virginity – and my self-respect

Some people say that too much masturbation, rushed masturbation at that, causes premature ejaculation. While this isn't true of everyone, I'm pretty sure that was at least partly to blame for me. When I was a kid, masturbation was very much a taboo subject and, like a lot of guys, I would rush it without giving it any thought.

I can't blame it all on that. I think some of it comes down to when I lost my virginity.

I was a bit of late starter, not losing my virginity until I reached the age of 19. I met the girl in a nightclub, she was a friend of a friend and, after the nightclub shut we headed back to my place to carry on with the fun we'd been having that night in the club.

Things heated up pretty quickly and, already pretty damn excited from the hours I'd spent dancing close with her, with all the flirting and the foreplay, we never even got close to having sex the first time – I was just too quick. At that point, I didn't know anything about premature ejaculation, had never even heard of it, but I did think that it would have been nicer to have lasted beyond zero seconds!

At the time I didn't realize it but, in that one single moment, my sexual confidence was knocked for six. In the way that many women do, she didn't let on how disappointed she as and, fair play to her, she tried so hard to make me feel that it was OK. Clearly, though, it wasn't.

Sadly, the second time was no better and, at that point, I was embarrassed and horrified, not just for me but for her too. What didn't occur to me was that this was the start of everything, the beginning of all my anxieties over performance.

And, just to add a bit more fuel to the fire, I now realize that my penis is physically sensitive – doomed from the start.

The excuses, the silence

To my shock and amazement, she stayed with me but over the next week or so, I found out how bad the problem really was. If I waited for 24 hours or more between sex sessions, I was done for, I couldn't last longer than a minute at the absolute most. If we had sex over and over again I would get better although I still never really managed to get over the five-minute mark. And that was only if she was prepared to wait for the third or fourth time that was a bit better.

As the months passed, our sexual relations got less and less. Do you know what the most shocking thing is, though? We never once talked about it – ever

To this day, the most embarrassing thing for me is that I never spoke to any partner about this problem over the next few years and I never did anything about it, either. Not even when I finally took the plunge and got married. Perhaps even worse is that none of my partners nor my wife ever mentioned it either. Well, my wife (now my ex-wife) would sometimes all me a "bastard", jokingly when I came too early.

To be fair, we would talk occasionally about the fact that I would come quickly on most occasions but we never talked about it in a way that would register it as a problem that needed to be fixed. All that happened is, like my first girlfriend, the sex got less and less to the point where it was a rare occurrence.

Selfishly, I turned the situation around and said that it happened because we didn't have sex very often and when we did, I just couldn't handle it. Whilst this is, in a small way, true, it doesn't change the fact that I should have sorted this problem sooner, that it was my problem, not hers.

Ironically, after I split up with my ex-wife (not because of the problems with sex), I could finally admit that I had a problem, a serious one that needed dealing with. The day I admitted it is a day I remember more clearly than the day I finally lost my virginity. It was an awful day as well as being a fantastic day. It was awful because, by admitting that I actually had this problem also made me realize that is should have admitted it sooner, many years sooner. I sat there and I thought about all the women I had left frustrated, screaming silently that I couldn't make it last. How many of them told their friends, people that I used to socialize with?

On the good side, the fact that I had finally acknowledged that I had a problem meant I could take steps to solve it.

Taking the first steps

As a man who spent so many years denying that I had a problem, ignoring it, when I finally did admit that is suffered from premature ejaculation, I suddenly found that I was extremely dedicated to solving the problem.

Obviously, the worst and hardest bit was in actually admitting that there was a problem. The rest, all the research and the steps in dealing with it, would be easy in comparison, or at least, I hoped they would. The first thing I did was searched the internet and read up on the subject in men's health publications but, sadly, I found most of the information was somewhat vague. Then I discovered a book called **The Ejaculation Trainer.**

That book was responsible for two things – it gave me hope ad it gave me homework to do. Apparently, the key to unlocking the problem of premature ejaculation is in practicing lots of different techniques while masturbating and/or having sex.

I discovered that there was no instant cure, that these techniques would pay off but not straight away. There were some tips that I could try straight away though and I did.

The next time I was lucky enough to have sex, I tried to use a number of the instant techniques and, yes, there were definitely a few improvements. It was hit and miss, though – sometimes I found I was lasting quite a bit longer while other times it was only a fraction longer.

The time I tried desensitization products

I never even knew these things existed until I read somewhere that you don't need to use them. Well, of course, that got my mind whirring. I already knew that I had a sensitive penis so it was worth a try, wasn't it?

The first one I tried was condoms impregnated with benzocaine – trust me guys, don't bother. Annoying isn't the word here. I tried a product called Priligy, but aside from the fact that it didn't really agree with me, it just didn't work.

I went on to try out a whole load of creams and sprays but, one after the other, they caused me problems or they just didn't work. The more I tried, the more frustrated I became because nothing seemed to work. Then I found a product called Promescent and, by god, it worked. Only as a temporary measure but it was a good one and, to my mind, a miracle.

So now I had this product that was helping me to last for between 10 and 20 minutes at a time, pretty good for the guy who never got past a couple of minutes before. Time to focus on the natural techniques I had learned to see if I could rid myself of this embarrassing and frustrating problem.

Natural techniques

For a couple of months, I stayed away from the women and kept to myself I needed time to get these techniques sorted and put them to the test. I practiced every single day and also learned to understand both my body and how to control my levels of arousal.

It must have been another two months before I was in a position to have sex again and I could put it all to the test. It was very difficult not to feel anxiety but it was important that I didn't. I had already done quite a bit of research about performance anxiety and I was fully prepared in having to deal with it; it seemed that all of the efforts I put in had paid off.

That first time again can't really be counted as a reliable marker because I'm ashamed to say, I was a little drunk, although this wasn't altogether a bad thing – alcohol does help me in that department! The next day when I had sex again was a different matter – I found that I could last much longer than I ever had before.

But, do you know what the most ironic thing about all of this is? I had come to realize that, by talking about it, the anxiety would be reduced and I would be able to last a lot longer. Believe me, the most awesome moment was when the woman I was with, the woman I had told about my problem, looked me in the eye and said, "trust me, you don't have a problem".

Could I at long last, say that I had overcome the problem of premature ejaculation?

It's an ongoing thing

What I came to understand is that, if these natural techniques were going to work forever I had to keep on doing them. If I slack off, my performance times drop, more so when I have been without a partner for a while and stayed away from women.

I have to regularly practice Kegel exercises or my strength starts to go, as does my control. I have to make sure that, whether I am with a partner or on my own, I take my time so I don't end going back to the bad habit of rushing.

If I chuck aside everything I learned about controlling my level of arousal, about breathing properly about learning when to stop, and all the other important things I learned, and just go at it, the difference in performance times just sucks. There is little I can do about it except for keeping up the techniques and the learning.

And, what doesn't help, I still have a sensitive penis; the likelihood is, it will probably always be that way and, I feel it is because of that, when I am with a new partner after being alone for a bit, that I still have problems.

In all honesty, that is when it is the most difficult to get all of the techniques I learned to work. So, when you have been without a partner for a while and you have had issues with premature ejaculation, it is important to be realistic in your expectation of how thing are going to be with a new partner, at least to start with.

The best advice I can give you

If it has suddenly occurred to you that you are not lasting as long as you should be in bed, the most important thing that must concentrate on is focusing your efforts on dealing with the problems. Don't do what I did, don't ignore it, the fact that you have a problem because it isn't going away. In fact, it will only get worse.

Do your research, find out exactly what works for you and never give up. The hardest part is n admitting that you have the problem in the first place; the rest, while not plain sailing, is considerably easier to deal with. Trial and error will play a big part in the next few months of your life but you will get there.

Now I can tell you something. I spent many years studying Psychology and I worked in mental health. So, how did it take me so many years to accept that I had a problem, that it was my responsibility and that I needed to deal with it? The point is, it doesn't matter who you are, it doesn't matter what you do as a job or what you study; the important thing is that you learn from my mistakes and don't ignore it,

Three years later

That was three years ago and, I am ecstatic to report, things are getting better by the day. A time has passed, I have learned to fully understand my body and levels of arousal; I can now determine when I get to the point of overheating and in danger of rushing things.

I can exert enough control over myself now to the stage where I can proudly say that I no longer suffer from the problem of premature ejaculation. 10 minutes or more are the norm for me now, on many occasions I can go for much longer.

Things take a step backward if I am in a high state of arousal and I don't use a condom but I now have a confidence I never had before; I can take full control of my sex life and I can do everything I need to keep things in check.

I don't use any kind of delay spray or desensitizing cream and over the years have come to realize that using natural techniques is the only way to deal with this.

Best advice? Don't hold back, get started on learning how you can control yourself today and learn how to last much longer in bed.

Many of the natural and other techniques that Sam used to help him are discussed throughout this book.

Bruce Maxwell

Chapter 4
Do's

Lasting long in bed will surely give every man a high. As he is able to satisfy his partner, his confidence is developed, and as he satisfies himself, he is living the sexual life he deserves. To deserve this erotic lifestyle, however, you must work hard and give importance to each of the factors affecting your poor performance.

Begin by keeping the end in mind. Do not lose sight of that goal. *The way to hours in bed and timely ejaculation may be long and challenging, but it can be done!*

Remember that the reproductive system and urinary system of a man work closely together; they even overlap at some instances. Caring for one is caring for the other—shooting two birds with one stone.

Protect your package!

A healthy tool will make a huge difference in your pursuit to last longer in bed. This means cleaning your tool every day with soap and water. If you are not circumcised, retract the foreskin to cleanse the penile head. This will minimize the risk of infection for you and your partner.

Avoid hurting your genital area. It is a very sensitive area and mechanisms in your reproductive system may get easily altered or damaged. Trauma like this may cause erectile dysfunction or premature ejaculation. Besides, you wouldn't want any anomalies threatening your genetic heritage, would you?

Avoid hot surfaces touching your scrotum. There is a reason your scrotum hangs way below your penile base. Very high temperatures may kill and/or dismember your sperm. It is like genocide for them.

Nature vs. Nurture

Give your package the nutrition it needs to perform its daily tasks with power. Eat balanced servings of protein, carbohydrates, and vegetables. Protein will ensure muscle growth and carbohydrates will give you the needed nutrients and energy to last longer in bed. Vegetables will ensure that there is enough oxygen carried in your blood to supply to the organs—especially your organ.

Drink fluids. Drink 1.5 to 2 liters of water daily. This does not include carbonated drinks, coffee, tea, and juices. This is to cleanse the urinary passage, which by the way, is also the road traveled by the semen when it shoots forth. This will also keep you hydrated during your coital adventures.

Urinate every 4 hours to keep your urinary tract clean. This will prevent you from contracting any infection in your most beloved part and leaving your partner an unwanted souvenir. Also, urinate before and after having sex. When an erection occurs, the valve that lets out urine closes. This causes urine to stagnate in your bladder, which may lead to bacterial proliferation. Lastly, bear down during urination to ensure that your bladder empties completely or at least has only a minimal amount of residue. This will prevent infection and thus, further damage to your tool.

17 Foods that Men Should Eat to Last Longer in Bed

Eating the right food is not just vital for your overall health; it can also help you to achieve much better performance in the bedroom department. You must eat foods that are full of the nutrients you need to promote good sexual health. Those nutrients are:

- Amino acids
- Niacin
- Phosphorus
- Potassium

- Vitamin-B complex
- Vitamin B6
- Vitamin B12
- Zinc

Provided you are feeding your body all of these vital nutrients, plus other vitamins and minerals, you can be sure that your performance will significantly improve over time and you can knock premature ejaculation on the head.

Poor diets are responsible for a lot of things, not least poor sexual performance, low levels of testosterone, a low quality of erection, no sex drive, impotence, no libido and premature ejaculation. Eating a good diet will clear up all of that and more, as well as helping you to last much longer in bed.

Think about that before you start popping pills and sing creams and sprays; sometimes all you need to do is change the way you eat.

So, what are these performance boosting foods then?

Leafy Green Vegetables

Eat plenty of these on a daily basis to increase your performance and improve your sexual health. Make sure you eat a good selection, including:

- Collards
- Kale
- Spinach
- Swiss chard
- Beet greens

Oatmeal

Oatmeal is a true power food, especially when it comes to sex. Eating oatmeal on a regular basis will provide you with a significant increase in energy levels and a boost in performance, helping you to stay the pace for a lot longer

Cereals

Eating a bowl of cereal at breakfast time will provide you with a range of the important nutrients you need. It will also help you to store energy for longer, resulting in a much better performance in bed

Nuts

Nuts should be a daily part of your diet to keep you healthy, active and energetic:

- Almonds
- Brazil nuts
- Butternuts

- Hazelnut
- Hickory nut
- Peanuts
- Pine nuts
- Pistachio
- Walnuts

All of these are packed full of powerful antioxidants and sex nutrients

Whole Grain

This is another fantastic food for helping to improve your stamina and improve your performance

Sunflower Seeds

These are perhaps the best of all the seeds, a real power food. Enjoy them on their own, on a salad, over a fish and vegetable meal, or you can blend them up in a sauce or a soup

Celery

Celery is a true powerhouse and you can eat it in a number of ways. Raw, add it to a salad or juice it with cucumber, spinach and lemon for a sexy smoothie. Try to drink one liter a day to really improve things in bed

Liver

Lamb and beef liver are full of B-vitamins and are extremely important for men and sex. They can help to increase your sperm count, your sexual desire, and your libido, as well as improving your performance

Steak

Steak contains a high level of sex nutrients making it one of the best foods to eat. It also raises the dopamine levels in your blood stream, helping you to be more aware of when you are about to ejaculate, giving you time to hold it back and get it under control

Salmon

Salmon is another good food for building up sexual stamina. They are full of nutrients and omega 3 fatty acid, providing you with everything you need for a top performance between the sheets

Oysters

The original aphrodisiac, the humble oyster is a true superhero for improving sexual health

Lobster

Lobster has long been linked to a healthy and strong male libido and is packed full of nutrients that can help to boost your sex drive and increase your sensitivity towards sex

Honey

Honey provides you with energy that will keep you on the go all night. Just add a spoonful or two of honey to a glass of milk and eat a handful of nuts before bed to give you plenty of energy and help you to last a lot longer in bed.

Dark Chocolate

Chocolate is actually good for you, provided you eat dark chocolate with a high cocoa content. It provides a boost to your energy levels but do watch how much you eat – it will quickly add calories to your diet

Yogurt

Eating a cup of yoghurt, nonfat variety, with a few blueberries provides you with one of the best sex foods of all time. Add a little of that honey to it and you will be raring to go – and keep on going. Try eating a yoghurt for breakfast, mixed with nuts and seeds as well

Ice Cream

Especially the good old vanilla flavor can increase your sex drive quite significantly. If you like to experiment with food during sex, you can't go wrong with vanilla ice cream. Not only will the smell work to relax you, your inhibitions will be lowered and you will have a much longer lasting power to keep going

Bananas

Eating bananas on a regular basis will give your sex life a real boost and provide you with lasting energy. They are packed full of potassium and Vitamin-B complex which are two of the most powerful of all the sex nutrients.

They won't stop you from having a premature ejaculation but they will give you the power to keep on going.

NOTE – Make sure you eat raw foods where you can and stick to organic. These contain the most nutrients, minerals and vitamins and have much less in the way of harmful chemicals.

So, there you go, 17 foods that are guaranteed to boost your sex life, increase your sex drive and help you to last longer in bed. Add in regular exercise and you will soon be seeing some fantastic change and sexual benefits

The Kegel Exercises

Do the Kegel exercise. It exercises the pubococcygeal muscle or the PC muscle by contracting it in a series of repetitions. Working on your PC muscle will give you more control on the progress of your intercourse. This helps you control premature ejaculation and gives you more intense pleasure during intercourse and orgasm.

Now that you know how to find your PC muscle (discussed in Chapter 2), you must make a religious effort to exercise at least 4 times a week. Do not do the Kegel exercises when your bladder is full! This may cause more harm as it weakens your supporting star rather than tone it. Furthermore, keep your buttocks, abdominal, and thigh muscles relaxed during the exercise to maximize the PC muscle contraction.

Beginners must start with doing the Kegel exercises sitting down. Find your PC muscle and contract it using a "drawing in" force. It is like holding in your urine. Hold it for 2 seconds. Do ten repetitions with 2-second intervals in between contractions. You may do 3 to 5 sessions a day.

After a couple of weeks doing beginner Kegel exercises, you may now move on to the intermediate level. Draw in your PC muscle for 5 seconds and relax it for another 5. Again, do this 10 times. Do 3 to 5 sessions a day.

As you progress to the advanced level, you will learn that your tolerance for contracting your PC muscle has increased significantly. You should now be able to hold your PC muscle in for 10 seconds and relax it for another 10. Do this 10 times in a session and do 5 to 8 sessions daily.

When you have mastered this, you may restart by doing the beginner exercises standing up. There is less support on your PC muscle this way, thus, it is worked out more intensely. Furthermore, when you feel that the advanced exercises done standing up post no more challenge to you, try doing the Kegel exercises with an erection. This should cause your penis and scrotum to move up and down. You may also do "Quickies." This is done by drawing in your PC muscle quickly and strongly 10 to 15 times.

During intercourse, mindfully doing the Kegel will cause intense friction that is not present during regular intercourse. It causes contractions, both in the vaginal canal and the penile shaft, which not only leads to orgasm but also enhances all sensory preceptors in the body. You will feel the sexual release not only in the genital area but also in the body's erotic zones. The nipples tickle, there is a warm feeling over the ears and the inner thighs contract.

Remember that you should only progress to the next level of exercises once you feel confident that you are stronger and able to tolerate more pressure. Work at your own pace and adjust the parameters to your abilities. You may alter the duration, interval, or repetition of the exercises to your liking. Keep in mind, however, that overworking your muscles may do more harm. Be very careful that you do not strain yourself.

Seeing the effect of such exercise is variable. It will depend on your conscious effort to exercise every day. When followed routinely, you should be able to contract your PC muscle for 10 seconds for 10 repetitions in about 3 to 4 months. There is no need to worry if you are behind schedule. As long as there has been some improvement, you will get to your goal with a little more work.

The Kegel exercises are easy to do and can be done anywhere as no actual movement can be seen from afar. *You can do it at work, while waiting for the bus, while on the subway on the way home, or even during an office meeting.* Do it diligently and you will be rightfully rewarded.

Use Toys

Modern times have made sex toys available and acceptable in the community. As you may use sex toys in the bedroom, some toys have been designed for strengthening the PC muscle. This is in the form of prostate massagers.

These are made basically for men with prostate problems such as enlargement and tumors. It works by inserting the massager into your anus. It doesn't need to go deep because even as you insert your finger into your anal canal, you may feel your prostate readily. As you contract your anal sphincter, the massager itself also contracts, serving the same purpose as the Kegel Exercises.

Tone Up

It is known that increased weight may cause erectile problems. So, you must exercise not only your PC muscle but your whole body as well.

Maintain your ideal weight. Circulation is impaired to areas with high densities of fat. Exercise will ensure that all your organs, including your most beloved organ, are supplied well with blood.

Running, swimming, biking, and other sports improve your stamina and agility. You can definitely use this for long, late hour frolicking. Your PC muscle may be in optimum condition but how do you last long in bed, when you tire easily?

Muscle toning workouts can also be useful in increasing strength, just in case you have to carry your woman through the house before putting her to bed.

Work on the core muscles so the PC doesn't have to do all the work. Crunches and deep lunges should ensure that the abdominal and thigh muscles can support your PC.

Take Matters Into Your Own Hands

Yes, I mean that once you recognize the problem, stand up and do something about it! And, yes, I also mean take some alone time and masturbate!

Practice is the key to learning how to control your urges. To avoid ending a hot, steamy session with your girl with a lot of apologies, you must practice!

Get to know yourself more, the sensations that easily make you excited and the circumstances that make you come early. Work with this knowledge to make each private meeting last longer.

Try the stop and start technique. Stimulate yourself up to the point near orgasm, but instead of ejaculating, stop. Let your body float back down to earth until you are stable and may start again. This will practice control.

Stress Release

Work, relationship and personal issues can take a toll on your body and thus, inhibit you from reaching your optimum sexual potentials. Release stress in a personalized activity that works for you.

You may watch primetime sitcoms or have some quality alone time with a book. You may attend Yoga classes or boxing if either of these suits you. You may spend a weekend at the beach or go to the karaoke bar with your friends. You could find a hobby you enjoy and reserve a couple of hours in a week for that sole purpose. Stick with whatever works for you.

You just have to be able to take some time out from life's stresses and anxieties.

Using Yoga to Help You Last Longer in Bed

While some men will turn their noses up at the thought of doing yoga, it is one of the best ways to ensure that you can last just that little bit longer in bed. The poses I am going to show you work by rejuvenating your body, regulating bodily functions and regulating hormone levels, with the result that your sex life is significantly improved as well.

Sarvangasana (Shoulder Stand)

This improves how your thyroid glands work to regulate the bodily functions, from an increase in metabolism to keeping your energy levels high through the whole day. The biggest and best effect of learning this asana is that it helps give your adrenal glands more strength, as well as strengthening up the way the testes work, thus giving your sperm and semen more potency. Here's how to do it:

- Lie down on a yoga mat and stretch your legs outwards
- Raise your legs slowly – you can do this by folding them in at the knees first or just by going for it and lifting them right up
- Support yourself with your palms by putting them on your hips and back, raising your body up while pointing your toes towards the ceiling. Keep all your weight on your shoulders and lock your chin to your chest. Breath slowly and make sure your elbows remain in contact with the floor and your back has support
- Hold for as long as you are comfortable
- Slowly lower your body back to the floor and back to your starting position. Do NOT just fall back to the floor as you could do some damage to your arms, shoulders and back

NOTE - This should not be attempted if you suffer from spinal injuries or neck injuries. If you are diagnosed with high blood pressure, this exercise should only be attempted under the supervision of a qualified person

Uttanapadasana (Raised Legs)

This is aimed at strengthening up your intestinal system. Ayurvedic principle maintains that the intestines are the key organ for a healthy body. This asana can also help to beat probes with digestion, constipation and to boost your metabolism. And, because it has such a good effect on your digestive system, this asana can also help you to control your ejaculation rate and beat premature ejaculation into submission. Here's how to do it:

- Lie on your yoga mat comfortably and put your hands to your sides; put your heels together
- Inhale deeply and raise your legs to 30-degree position at the same time as raising your head from the floor
- Hold for just a few seconds and then slowly take your legs and head back down to the floor
- Repeat but this time, raise your legs up to 60 degrees
- If you struggle to lift both legs at the same time, just do one at a time. It won't take long before you are flexible enough to do both at the same time

NOTE - If you suffer from knee or back injuries/pain, this asana should only be done under the supervision of a qualified instructor

Kandharasana (Shoulder Pose)

This is a fantastic asana for increasing the sexual desire of both men and women. Aside from the fact that it can help to strengthen up the sperm in a man and the ovaries in a woman, it can also help couples who are infertile. On top of this, it can help to clear up menstrual disorders, discharge that comes from infections and increases the amount of lubrication in the vagina. Here's how to do it:

- Lie flat on your yoga mat
- Bend your knees until your ankles are resting against your buttocks
- Keep your legs separated slightly
- Grab your ankles, inhale and then hold your breath
- Raise your buttocks into the air slowly and push your chest upwards
- At this point, you should have an arched back
- Hold for as long as you can
- Return to the floor by exhaling and lowering down slowly

NOTE - If you are diagnosed with high blood pressure, or suffer from any spinal disorders or pain in the lower back, only do this asana under the guidance of a qualified instructor

Paschimotasana (Seated Forward Bend)

This is by far the best asana if you are looking to beat premature ejaculation and last longer in bed. It is also useful for helping to make semen more potent by strengthening up the perm. On top of that, it is a great metabolism booster. Here's how to do it:

- Sit up straight, your legs closed together and stretched out. Your feet should be pointing towards the ceiling

- Inhale deeply and stretch your arms up
- Exhale and bend forwards, keeping your spine straight and erect
- Grab the big toes on your feet between your thumb and index finger, breathing in while you do this
- Exhale and bend forwards gradually so that your forehead touches your knees and your elbows touch the floor beside you
- Hold this position for 10 to 20 seconds as a minimum holding your breath
- Inhale and go slowly back to your starting position
- Repeat five or six times to gain the benefits of the asana

Note - If you suffer from pain in the back or problems with the spine, do NOT do this asana as it could make things much worse.

You may find it hard to touch your forehead to your knees to start with. Go as far as you can without causing yourself any pain and keep on practicing. The more you do it, the more flexible you will become.

Goumukhasana (Cow Head Pose)

This is a good asana to help fix a hernia and with hydrocele which is a buildup of fluid in the testes. It can also help in controlling the rate of ejaculation very effectively, as well as strengthening up the liver, respiratory system and the kidneys. Here's how to do it:

You should do this with all your weight on your knees if you can. However, if you can't or you have arthritis that stops you from doing it, you can sit to do it. To do it the right way, on your knees:

- Kneel on your yoga mat, keeping your back and upper body straight and your weight squarely on your knees
- Keep your toes pointing down and into the ground
- Bend your right arm at the elbow and put it behind you, keeping your fingertips facing up and close to your spine
- Raise your left arm above your head, bending it at the elbow again
- Place it on the nape of your next and try to grasp it with your right hand
- Breathe as you would normally
- To return to your starting position, sit down slowly and then take your hands back to the starting position

NOTE – If you find that you cannot grasp your hands together, don't worry. As you practice, you will gain flexibility and will find it much easier to do

Bhujangasana (Cobra Pose)

This is an excellent asana for healing both cervical and back pain, as well being highly effective in helping you to last longer in bed and help to address premature ejaculation. Here's how to do it:

- Lie flat on your yoga mat on your stomach
- Make sure your feet are stretched flat to the floor and put your forehead to the floor
- Put your hands, palms down, on the floor beside your shoulders, keeping your elbows as close to your body as you can – they must not flare outwards
- Exhale and lift up your upper body, a little at a tie – head first, then chest, back and, lastly, pelvis
- Your hands should be straight and your elbows locked. Your navel must be touching the floor and equal pressure is placed on both hands
- Breathe in and breathe out slowly, calming your mind
- To get out of this asana, breath out and slowly lower yourself back down to a lying position
- To sit up, turn onto your side and use your palms to help you up

NOTE - If you suffer from pain or injury to the wrist or back, do not do this asana – also not for pregnant women

Dhanurasana (Bow Pose)

This asana is well known for helping a person to have a much stronger orgasm, as well as helping to beat premature ejaculation. It is also good for healing stomach problems. Here's how to do it:

- Lie on your yoga mat, on your stomach, with your feet placed at a hip's width apart
- Your arms should be beside your body
- Fold your knees upwards and grab your ankles
- Breathe in, lift up your chest, off the ground, and pull your legs back and upwards
- Look ahead of you and smile
- Hold this pose while focusing on your breathing and keep taking deep breaths
- Do not overdo this, it is easy to get carried away. Hold it for a maximum of 15 to 20 seconds
- Exhale, lower your legs and chest gently back to the ground and let go of your ankles
- Relax

NOTE - You should not do this asana is if you have been diagnosed with either low or high blood pressure, a hernia, injury or pain to the neck or lower back, migraine, headache or have had surgery on your stomach recently – also not for pregnant women

Brahmacharyasana (Celibate's Pose)

This is an excellent asana for people who repeatedly suffer from nightfall and a decrease in excitement sexually. If can also help to regulate how the testes work and help the digestive system. Here's how to do it:

- Kneel on your yoga mat, keeping your feet apart slightly
- Make sure your knees touch each other and your feet are pointing out
- Lower your body very slowly into the space in between your legs
- Make sure your buttocks are touching on the floor and put your palms on your knees, face down
- Breathe normally and shut your eyes so you can concentrate properly
- Hold for a few minutes and then reverse the process to get back to your starting position

NOTE - Do not do this asana if you have any problems with your knees or with any other injury

Garudasana (Eagle Pose)

This asana helps to relieve any issues that are related to the prostate gland, testes and to help in premature ejaculation. It is also good for helping to relieve any symptoms associated with diseases of the reproductive system and urinary tract. Here's how to do it:

First, you must learn the Tadasana pose:

- Stand on your yoga at with your arms by your side and your feet together

- Make sure the weight is even across the arches and the balls of your feet
- Breathe in a steady rhythm and be aware of your inner self
- Focus only on now, pushing all your worries to one side
- Press the big toes together, pushing your heels apart if you need to
- Raise your toes and spread the out, then, one at a time, put them down on the mat
- If you can't balance, place your feet about six inches apart
- Straighten your leg, drawing down through your heels
- Make sure your feet are firmly grounded and press down evenly across the four corners of each foot
- Lift up your ankles and arches, squeezing the outer shins in towards each other
- Engage your quadriceps, drawing the top of your thighs up and back at the same time
- Slightly rotate your thighs so they face inwards and widen out your sit bones
- Pull your tailbone in a little but make sure you do not round out your back
- Raise the back of your thighs releasing your buttocks and keep your hips in line with the center of your body

- Put your pelvis into a neutral position, making sure your hip bones are pointing straight ahead, not up or down. Draw in your belly a little
- Inhale, elongating your torso
- Exhale releasing your shoulder blades down towards your waist
- Keep your shoulders lined up the side of your body and broaden your collarbones
- Press your shoulder blades down towards the back of your ribs but make sure you do not squeeze them in together
- Make sure your arms stay straight, your finger should be extended and your triceps held firm
- Let your inner arms turn slightly outwards
- Stretch your neck keeping your shoulders, ears, hips ad ankle in lie with each other
- Breathe evenly and smoothly
- Each time you exhale, you should feel your spine begin to elongate
- Gaze forwards and hold for up to a minute

Once you have mastered this pose, you can move on to the Garudasana:

- Stand in the above position on your yoga mat

- Bend your right leg slightly at the knee, placing all of your weight onto it
- Lift up your left leg and wrap it around the other, pressing your left foot against your right calf
- Raise up your hand in front, holding them parallel to the floor
- Bend your right elbow
- Wrap your left hand around it making sure that both of your palms face each other
- Hold the position for a few seconds and then return slowly to your starting position

NOTE - This asana is difficult and will take a great deal of concentration. Practice really does make perfect. Although you may fall the first couple of times you do it, the more you practice, the longer you will be able to hold the pose

Anulom Vilom Pranayam

This is more of a breathing technique that has been shown to help a few problems, like allergies of the respiratory system, colds, coughs, sinusitis, and rhinitis. However, it can also help to improve sexual pleasure and make your orgasms feel much better and stronger, as well as helping to slow down the rate of ejaculation. It also gives your entire body strength. Here's how to do it:

- Sit on your yoga mat and cross your legs. Try to fold your knees as completely as you can; if not, just go as far as you can without causing any pain or injury. If you suffer from arthritis, you can do this while sitting on a straight-backed wooden chair

- Turn one hand so your palm faces upwards. With the other hand, place your thumb against one nostril and fold in the index finger

- Keeping your ring finger extended out, use it to close the other nostril

- Make sure your elbow is not held too high because your hand will get tired too quickly

- Inhale through one nostril, keeping your finger on the other to keep it closed

- Open the other nostril and shut the one you breathed through last – exhale. This will be one cycle

- Breathe in and repeat the above process

- Practice for about 3 minutes to start with but do increase your time up to about 15 or 20 minutes

- Remember, you mustn't raise your shoulders, or slouch them when you breathe in. Use your lungs to breathe in deeply, not just your stomach

Practice these poses regularly to increase libido, beat premature ejaculation and last a lot longer in bed.

Bruce Maxwell

Issues Kill the Buzz

Health: Check. PC muscle: Check. Exercise: Check. Practice: Check. But, you are still having problems! Do remember that premature ejaculation is a multi-factorial occurrence. Check all your bases first before running out into the world saying that you have a medical problem.

Make sure that you are comfortable with what you are doing, and that your partner is, too. Problems in your relationship may cause enough stress to give you problems in the sack. So, check this!

Talking to your partner and working on the situation together, be it the relationship or the problems in bed, may help tremendously in gaining control of the beast that consumes you in the bedroom.

Doctor, Doctor

If any other matter still concerns, confuses, and troubles you, any doctor will not hesitate to help you. For psychosocial problems, you may visit a therapist alone or with your partner. For physical problems, you may also get tested and treated. Do not hesitate to ask for help.

5 Shocking Things That Can Help You Last Longer in Bed

If there are two things that most men are insecure about, whether they admit it or not, it is sex and the size of their penis. All men, no matter what walk of life they come from, like to be proud of the size of their lunchbox and of how long they can last in bed, simply because they are of the belief that a bigger than average size and the ability to last much longer are the two things that build up the sexual appetite of the woman they are with. Unfortunately, there is little they can do about the size of their tools, they can do something to make themselves last a god deal longer in bed.

While it can be an advantage in some things to be able to finish quickly, sex is not one of them. In fact, premature ejaculation is one of the most common of all the sexual problems that a man suffers from and is also the most distressing for both parties. Recent research found that an immense 45% of men finish too quickly, within two minutes of starting sex. The average time for sex is 7.3 minutes, about 4 minutes less than the average woman would like it to last.

OK, so this is probably quite discouraging for both men and women but it is important to remember that both stamina and performance can be enhanced and improved in some unlikely ways. Here are just five of those ways:

1. **A big belly**

Contrary to what you have been told, size really does matter in terms of sex. Unfortunately, it isn't the size of your tool, it is the size of your belly. A study published in 2010 in The Journal of Sexual Medicine, said that men with bigger bellies made better lovers. Men who were overweight, with an obviously larger belly, were lasting the average of 7.3 minutes while thinner men could hardly make it to the two-minute mark. This might seem to be somewhat counterintuitive but, the research determined that the more belly fat a man has, the higher the level of estradiol, which is the female sex hormone, and this is what helps to slow the orgasm down.

2. **Adult Circumcision**

We've all heard the phrase, "better late than never", and we all know that it can apply in a number of different ways, and that includes adult circumcision. In 204, a study that was published in the Adult Urology journal revealed that men who were circumcised took quite a bit longer to ejaculate, after being circumcised as an adult. While some people will believe this to be a hindrance, there are those, particularly those who suffer from premature ejaculation, who will see this as a blessing. The study originated in the GATA Haydarpasa Training Hospital in Istanbul and was carried out by urologist Temucin Senkul. He determined that the delay was down to the circumcision having an effect on penis sensitivity

3. **Exercise – Pelvic Floor**

These exercises are not just for women or for people who have problems with their bladder; they can also be of great help in treating premature ejaculation. The European Congress of Urology in Stockholm carried out a study on 40 men, aged between 19 and 46, who averaged 31.7 seconds for ejaculation. They were set 12 weeks of pelvic floor exercises and, at the end, 33 of the men showed a marked improvement in ejaculation time along with a significant increase in self-confidence. By the end of the 12 weeks, the average time had risen to 146.2 seconds, almost four times what it was at the start of the research.

4. **A Vegetarian Diet**

If there is one thing that staunch vegetarians are known for, it is the strength of the stance they take on dairy and meat intake. However, they are also known for being able to last longer in bed, because of an increase in both energy and stamina. Vegan diets, high in fruit, can give you a much higher level of sustainable energy, that will not be subject to the "sugar crash" that we often see with a typical western diet packed full of processed sugars. Bananas, for example, are very high in potassium, which is a nutrient helpful to the production of sex hormones and for boosting energy levels.

Various and numerous tests have shown that those who eat a vegetarian diet have got twice the level of stamina than a meat eater. The Yale medical Journal published a study that compared athletes who ate meat to athletes who were vegetarian or near-vegetarian – half of these latter groups led a sedentary lifestyle. The research involved measuring how long each person in the study could hold their arms outstretched and how many deep knee bends they could do. Just 13% of the meat eaters could keep their arms outstretched for 15 minutes, compared to a whopping 69% of vegetarians. None of the meat eaters could keep their arms out for 30 minutes while 4% of the vegetarians could. With the knee bends, 33% of meat eaters managed more than 352, against 81% of the vegetarians.

5. **Viagra**

The famous little blue pill. While it was mainly used to treat impotence or erectile dysfunction, it also has its uses when it comes to giving the sexual performance a boost. The magic ingredients in Viagra are phosphodiesterase-5 inhibitors, female hormones that delay orgasm. A 2012 study that was published in the Journal of Sexual Medicine showed that the pill could help men to extend the lime they lasted in bed before they had an orgasm.

Out of 14 studies, 11 of them showed that the medication could be associated with lasting longer in bed but not all of the studies could say for definite if Viagra was the responsible ingredient as it was never tested against anything else, most specifically a placebo.

When it comes to premature ejaculation, the key to beating it, or to improving your sexual stamina, can be down to something as simple as mind over matter. Athletes have to practice hard to increase their stamina and their energy levels and the same is true of sex. At the end of the day, there isn't a problem that can't be got over so get practicing.

Bruce Maxwell

Chapter 5
Don'ts

Being the best lover also entails you to make many sacrifices. You will also need to identify which are the right sacrifices to make. In this chapter, you will learn the right things to avoid so that you will last longer in bed.

Tobacco and alcohol do not help you in any way in bed. As a matter of fact, both these vices cause premature death of cells in the body. You will feel more tired and will contract illnesses easily. Furthermore, abnormalities in sperm have been found in men taking large amounts of alcohol and smoking pack after pack of cigarettes daily. It may give you a temporary sexual boost, but when taken collectively, a part of your manhood dies every day with each intake.

Men wanting to last longer in bed must also avoid drugs. Medication for certain illnesses such as anti-depressants and antibiotics may cause your reproductive mechanism to be altered. Avoid getting sick and ask your doctor if there are any possible side effects when taking medications. He should also inform you of what should be done about these side effects or you may ask for an alternate drug which has fewer adverse effects.

Do not use commercial drugs. Long-term use may cause irreparable damage not only to your reproductive parts but to your performance as well. They may alter your hormonal compositions and sperm-making abilities.

In fact, the only drugs you should be using are those prescribed by your doctor for the treatment of chronic premature ejaculation. Drugs have more than a few drawbacks, especial the chemical options. Even prescribed drugs can affect your ability to have an orgasm, with some people finding that they can't orgasm at all, no matter how much they want to.

Do not use desensitizing creams. They are meant to desensitize your shaft to make the sex act longer without premature ejaculation. This, however, diverts the whole purpose of sex. Sex should be a sensory activity, where the male and female share the pleasure. Even worse, when you rub off the cream to your partner, now, both you will be feeling no sensations—so much for lasting long in bed. So, stay organic!

Also, avoid thinking of "un-sexy" things while getting it on. Many use this diversion to delay their ejaculation. This, however, only causes more sexual problems as you are not able to participate in the act as deeply as you should. This will also bring forth more psychological problems in the future.

It's an old thought that you can stop yourself from coming by thinking of something totally unerotic but that is a really old misconception. As a starter, premature ejaculation is normally caused by anxiety, not by how turned on you feel. By thinking of something else and trying to distract yourself, you are only placing more emphasis on how anxious you really are. And that, my friends, is the total opposite of what you are supposed to be achieving.

One of the biggest parts about controlling your body is learning how to be aware of it, not distracting yourself. The more aware you are of what triggers and sensations your body feel while you are having sex, the easier you will be able to learn how to control them and how to respond to them.

Anyway, the point of sex is to be with your partner, not distracting yourself right at the moment so you are paying them no attention whatsoever. If your mind is distracted, it shows and they will know about it. That's just a little bit insulting to them and is not helping you in the slightest.

Before we take things any further, let's just look at something else, something which has a direct bearing on everything you have read and what you are about to read.

The Difference between a Problem and a Preference

This really is one of the very first issues to address – what is the difference between a real problem, like premature ejaculation, and someone saying "I can't last as long as I would like". One of these is a preference, not a problem while the other is a real issue that often requires medical intervention to solve it. We know that premature ejaculation is defined as "a persistent or recurring uncontrolled ejaculation" and we know that it tends to happen either before or within one minute of penetration happening. It also happens before either partner is ready. Sadly, for the people involved, it is the most common of all the sexual dysfunction, with more than a third of men surveyed, aged 18 to 59, reporting that it happened regularly.

Somehow, it isn't any comfort to hear the words, "don't worry, it happens to lots of people". The trickiest thing about this problem is that there isn't one single cause that you can pinpoint. It is a mixture – anxiety learned behavior and overstimulation. Chronic cases may require professional assistance to get to the bottom of it. However, while it is a very real problem for some men, the real issues lies in the idea that real men can "bang away" for hours before they even feel the need to have an orgasm – never mind the poor woman underneath you! That is the biggest problem You see, there are quite a few people who believe that penetration has to be for at least 30 minutes, the actual average time is seven minutes, with between three and five being seen as adequate and anything lower as a real problem. Nobody wants to be "adequate" and certainly none of you wants to be in the problem category so how can we improve things between the sheets? Here is one more major don't for you:

Don't watch any more porn

One of the biggest problems with anxiety about staying power is, sadly, down to porn. This is because most sex education tends to focus primarily on anatomy and on sexually transmitted diseases, doing nothing whatsoever to talk about sexual pleasure, potency, and virility. Most of that kind of education comes from porn and that causes a real issue – porn bears absolutely no resemblance to real sex.

Porn is all about looking right on the camera, not what feels right and that means we learn all the wrong lessons. That means we watch these marathon sessions between porn stars and think that we should be able to last that long. Get it into your head – porn is fake. They don't really last that long; most of the scenes are edited together, making you believe you are watching one session instead of the several that it really is. The men in these films use numbing agents, or, believe it or not, they pull out, slapping their tools against their partner's thigh or vagina to stop themselves from ejaculating.

Not only that, think about your poor woman! She doesn't want you slamming into her for hours – that's going to hurt!

Chapter 6

Five Positions to Help You Last Longer in Bed

Women tend to take longer to become aroused and reach orgasm than men do and this can create more than a few problems in the bedroom department. It really doesn't have to, though. If you want to stay the distance, try these top five sex positions, all designed to hold your arousal back and last longer, ending with both of you being satisfied.

Make sure that you indulge in lots of foreplay and introduce sex games to try and spice it up a little. This can help to make sure both of you are relaxed, excited and are enjoying the sex. Follow up with one or more of these positions to prolong the pleasure for both of you.

1. **Cross**

This is something of a tricky position to get into because it requires you to lay on your side facing your woman while she lay on her back, with her legs draped over your pelvis, perpendicular to you. When you are both in a comfortable position, penetrate her; she will need to open her legs and push against you. The real beauty of the cross position is that the penetration goes quite a bit deeper than other positions and that works to enhance the pleasure on both sides. Because you are on your side, you won't be able to move so much and you won't be able to get carried away too quickly.

2. **Spooning**

For this position, you both need to lay on your sides, both of facing the same way. You will be, obviously, behind her and will be able to gently penetrate her, using slow rocking motions as your bodies get together. This is only going to allow for a shallow penetration so you should last quite a bit longer because you won't get overstimulated. And the slower motion of this position should feel fantastic for both of you. You could wrap your arms around her to give a deeper feeling of intimacy, a vital part of great sex.

3. **Doggy**

Perhaps this is one of your partner's favorite positions but it gets you excited so quickly you can't hold back. That' easily remedied with one simple change. Begin as you would normally for the doggy position -your partner on her hands and knees and you kneeling behind her, crouched over the top of her. Penetrate her and, as you do, she should lower her body slowly until she is lying flat on her stomach. Follow her down, keeping up with the movements so you stay in her and then either lie directly on top of her or hold yourself slightly off her on your knees. This will stop you from getting stimulated too quickly and you will both still get the full pleasure from the position.

4. **Sitting**

This can be quite a comfortable position. You sit cross-legged and your partner sits on you, facing you, with her legs wrapped around your back and her arms line around your neck to give a deeper intimacy. With rocking motions that are gentle, this position can be held for a long time. It is slow, it is passionate and it gives you the opportunity for deep penetration without becoming too excited, too quickly.

5. **On Top**

To be in total control of your session, your woman needs to be on top. This gives you very deep penetration and a nice view to look at and she gets to determine the pace. Your woman can lean forward a little and rest on her elbows to make the ecstasy last longer and you get a better chance of hitting her G-spot as well but without the aggressive thrusting of some other positions. This position also allows for more intimacy.

Bruce Maxwell

Chapter 7
Go Forth and Hone Your Skills!

Women are complex creatures designed by God to confuse men. It is difficult to tell what they want because they themselves do not know what they want.

If you are on a date, what you say now may make you a man she despises tomorrow, when she has had more time to think about it; your kind gesture she may find annoying in a moment's snap; and your gentleman's ways she may see as weak in the blink of an eye. She may change her point of view about a topic you have discussed without much reason and say that you really just don't have chemistry.

She may be able to make up endless excuses just so she won't have to see you again, but if you were good in bed, she might just give you another chance.

Dating and relationships are not all about sex, but really? What woman could resist a man that could make her roll her eyes back and grit her teeth?

Women claim to have intuition, but what they really have is an ability to read a person. She can tell how confident you are at dinner, when you tell stories about work or when you answer her questions about your family. She can feel the sexual tension you exude while watching a movie. She can feel you still when her hair brushes your ear. She will notice every little action, every little word you say and from this, she can judge easily.

So do yourself—and the women out there waiting for you—a favor. Before you go out into the world, make sure that your gun is fully loaded and ready to shoot. Clean yourself up, be healthy, groom yourself to take on the challenge, and be sure you have had practice!

When you are confident about yourself, that confidence shines through and is felt by other people, and that is just the key. People say that lasting long in bed gives you confidence. I believe it does. However, I also believe that confidence makes you last longer in bed.

Reading this book is only a pinch of what you have to do. Now that you have the knowledge, you will have to act on it. May this book serve as one of your life's manuals. Share it with the world and help your fellowmen as it has helped you. Share it with your partner, and you shall reap the benefits.

Bruce Maxwell

Chapter 8

16 Top Ways to Make You Last Longer in Bed

So, this is more of a recap with a few new ideas thrown in for good measure. At the end of the day, most men want to be able to last longer in bed, not just those who suffer from premature ejaculation. We all know it isn't any fun for either of you when things end too quickly but, on the other hand, all the media hype that says you should be going at it for half an hour or more is also wrong. Many men are conscious of the fact that they may be finishing just a little too quickly for their partner as all those Hollywood movies and magazines would have you believe women love sessions that go on for hours.

That is all complete and utter rubbish and nothing but hype. That said, there are times when you could do with lasting just a little longer than a few minutes so here are some killer tips to help you hold back for longer:

1. **Back to your teenage years**

Remember how, as a teenager, you used to spend what felt like hours kissing and making out without actually having sex? Felt good, didn't it. So, go back to doing that. Spend more time on kissing your partner, on exploring each other using your hands and your mouth before you even think about actually having sex

2. **Learn how to massage**

When you lead a busy life, it becomes quite difficult to find the time for sex and it isn't easy to make the move from your busy working life to a sexy erotic one. Stress is the culprit here and before you can even begin to feel like getting down to it, you need to de-stress. The very best way to do that is through massage, and if you do it properly, both you and your partner will be completely turned on by it. You do need to learn how to do this properly though; if you don't you can actually cause more problems. Learn to give a very deep and satisfying massage and then each of you takes about 5 or 10 minutes to massage each other before you think about sex. Not only are you really getting in the mood but you will be helping each other to breathe properly and to relax Foot and back messages are perfect for priming you for pleasure and comfort and, think of it this way – each minute you spend intimately massaging your partner is another minute towards your goal of lasting longer in bed.

3. **Take it in turns**

Most sexual sessions are pretty much a give and take pleasure method, in which each of you touches each other at the same time, which means you are both heading for the finish line pretty darn quick. There is a golden rule here if you really want things to take longer – take it in turns to touch each other. From now on, let your partner do the touching while you relax, lie back and take as much pleasure from it as you can without getting too over-excited. Then return the favor; let her lie back while you do the touching and exploring. Both of you need to learn how to use your hands properly to give as much pleasure as possible, leading both of you down the road to arousal but not so quick as it would normally happen.

4. **Control your surroundings**

The truth of the matter is when you are in a comfortable position, in comfortable surroundings, a place where either you or your partner is likely to get too over excited, you are more likely to last longer in bed. Don't be tempted with public sex or anything else that could be just that little too exciting for you. If your most comfortable place for sex is in bed then keep it in the bedroom, at least until you have learned how to control your orgasm.

5. **Woman on top**

I mentioned this one earlier; by having the woman on top, you don't feel so stimulated. Plus, ask her to take it slowly. Long, hard and fast thrusts are pretty dangerous for a man on the edge! You could also try penetrating her and then not moving for a couple of minutes, just to let yourself get acclimatized to her.

6. **Use the start-stop technique**

With this technique, your woman will stimulate you until you start to get close to an orgasm. At this point, tell her that she must stop. When your levels of sexual tension have reduced, it could be as quick as 15 seconds, start again. By doing this frequently, not only will you last longer for that particular session but you will also begin to understand your own feelings and will learn how to stop yourself.

7. **Learn to breathe from the belly**

When you breathe deeply, it is actually a direct correlation to ejaculation. So, breathing deeply and slowly should help you to reduce the stress and the anxiety, thus slowing down your rate of ejaculation. Learn how to breathe so that your belly will rise before your chest does and practice this in conjunction with the start-stop technique. You could also practice the yoga breathing technique I told you about earlier.

8. **Read the Kama Sutra**

Preferably together as this will heighten the pleasure for both of you. Plus, you could always try out some of the positions! In all seriousness, though, there is a specific technique that is mentioned that can help you to stay the distance. Using this technique, start off very slowly, with just one in and out stroke per three seconds. Then you can begin to build up the strokes, adding in more, over a session of about four or five minutes until you are at the stage where you are giving one stroke per second. If you feel as if you are about to lose control, stop, stay inside your woman until you regain control and then start from the beginning again

9. **Out of your head**

And I do not mean on drugs or alcohol! One of the biggest killers during sex, the one thing that will affect whether you can maintain an erection or not, is stress. And that comes down to what is going through your mind. In the case of premature ejaculation or in those who seem to rush it all the time, the main thoughts are going to be on your abilities and your performance and that will likely push you over the edge. Learn how to change your thinking to positivity and confidence pushing worry and stress out of the way. If you start to feel anxious or stressed during sex, stop, breathe deeply and then focus on your inner self. Get rid of the negative thoughts and put your attention firmly on you and your feelings.

10. **Try new positions**

I gave you five positions to try earlier to help you last longer in bed but you could always open that copy of the Kama Sutra. There are specific positions that are designed to make your orgasm happen quicker and others, like the ones I told you about that will prolong things. Experiment, try a few out and see what works and what doesn't.

11. **Learn to control your ejaculatory muscle**

When you ejaculate, do you ever wonder what physically causes it to happen? There is a specific muscle that controls your ejaculation and, when it is relaxed, you simply cannot ejaculate, no matter how hard you try. We talked about it earlier – it's called the PC muscle and it what is responsible for letting the semen come out when you come. To control your rate of ejaculation, you have to know how to control this muscle. Practice the exercises we talked about earlier as much as you can until you have almost full control over it. This won't be instant; it can take as much as four weeks to get really good results. It will also take a great deal of regular practice to get it right and become a sexual master.

12. **Learn to control your confidence and mental health**

Back in the olden days, it used to be thought that premature ejaculation was the result of mental health problems and men who suffered with it were immediately sent for hypnotherapy or to see a psychiatrist. Obviously neither of those worked very well. While premature ejaculation is a physical condition, it is also linked to mental health and this must not be ignored. You must learn how to manage your concentration levels, your thoughts, and your confidence levels while you are having sex. If you don't, it will have a serious effect on how long you can manage to last for.

13. **Masturbate often**

If you truly want to know how to last a long as possible between the sheets, you need to get more in tune with your own sexual responses. To do that, you're going to have to masturbate more. When you begin to stimulate yourself, make sure that you stop before you can't. Let's say that, on a scale of 1 to 10, the orgasm is number 10. So stop yourself at about 8. Make sure you leave time to calm down and then start again, working your way back up that scale. Do this as often as you need to in order to learn how to control yourself.

14. **Learn how to cool down**

Whether you suffer from premature ejaculation or not, you should till learn a few methods for cooling down. You can practice these so that, if you do find yourself heading towards being out of control you can stop yourself before you do go over the edge. Do your research and find the methods that will work for you, that will help you to last a bit longer in bed.

15. **Change it up**

What is the absolute best thing you can do when you find yourself heading fast toward that point of no return? The biggest piece of advice that I can give you is to change your speed. Men should have a go at teasing their partners; remove your tool from inside her and rub the head up and down over her sex. There are a lot of nerve endings there and this will make her feel great, as well as help to slow you down a bit.

16. **Squeeze**

Earlier on, we mentioned the most sensitive parts of the penis. There are three areas that, when squeezed, can help to slow you down and keep you hard. First, when your penis is erect, make a ring wth your index finger and your thumb around the base of it and squeeze it. This stimulates a ring around the base of the penis which helps to keep the blood where it should be. The second place is underneath the head of the penis. Applying pressure there can work wonders as it is the hot spot in most men and is full of nerve endings. Lastly, the perineum, the spot that is located in between the anus and the base of your testicles.

All of these techniques are designed for you, with you in mind. Obviously, you don't need to do all of what you have learned in this book, just what you feel comfortable doing, what makes you and your partner feel good and what works. Basically, do whatever it takes to make your bedtime sessions last as long as you both want them to.

There is something here that I must reiterate. You may think that it is OK to go for hours in bed and that may be what you are aiming for. Please don't. Unless your partner is a machine or made of some other substance than blood, skin and bone, it isn't wise or pleasurable to make sex last for a prolonged period of time, especially not the penetration part of it. It can be painful and uncomfortable, not just for your woman but for you too. Too much thrusting away can cause lubrication to dry up and then it become less of the pleasure and much more of the pain. You aren't in the movies and you don't need to perform for the cameras, just for you and her.

Bruce Maxwell

Conclusion

I hope that this book has been able to help you to maximize your lover skills; as I mentioned in the introduction, you must commit to performing the exercises which have been presented to you. There isn't any other way to get the result that you and your woman need.

For men who suffer from premature ejaculation, it will probably take some time to get yourself to a stage where you can control your orgasm and control yourself. You have to learn to understand your own body and your own mind first, before you can even begin to think about lasting any longer in bed. Take heart from Sam's story – it might have taken him some time to get there but he did. Also remember that, three years on, he is still having to keep up his exercises and all the methods that he learned to increase is staying power. And, don't forget what he taught you, what you need to learn from. Premature ejaculation is not something to be ignored and brushed aside. It won't get any better; indeed, it will actually get worse so man up and do something about it because, if you don't, you will go through life getting more and more stressed out without truly understanding where you have gone wrong.

It isn't a case of learn it once, do it twice and then forget about it. Stamina takes time to build up and it takes more than just a few minutes each day to do it as well. Diet plays a very important part as it affects your overall health and wellbeing. As you have seen, eating the right kinds of food can have incredible results on both the strength of your erection, and your staying power.

Learn new techniques for pleasuring both yourself and your woman in bed. Things like massage, and sex games can spice up your love life no end and can also help you to hold back a little, only letting go when you are both ready.

Remember that all of us deserve to enjoy life's pleasures to the maximum, and you are about to reach that goal on the sexual plane

Finally, if you enjoyed this book, please take the time to share your thoughts and post a review on Amazon. It'd be greatly appreciated!

Thank you and good luck!

Check Out My Other Books

Below you'll find some of my other popular books that are popular on Amazon and Kindle as well. I have added some other books from fellow authors in order to support their job too.

Simply search them on Amazon Kindle by the Title below to check them out. Alternatively, you can visit my author page on Amazon to see other work done by me.

- **Positive Thinking Works!**

Become happier and fearless learning how to change your thoughts positively!

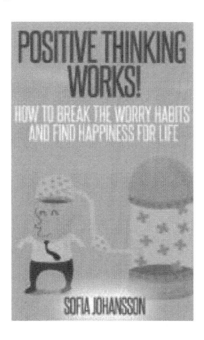

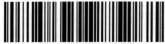

Made in the USA
Columbia, SC
24 November 2018